GYMBAG WISDOM
106 Ways To Become A Better Athlete

by

ZonePress
Doylestown, PA

GYMBAG WISDOM
106 Ways To Become A Better Athlete
(Physically, Mentally, and Emotionally)

A special thanks to Lisa.

Copyright © 2002 ZonePress

No part of this publication may be used or reproduced in any manner whatsoever without written permission of the publisher.

1st Edition

Design, Illustration, & Production: Ampersand Design, Inc., Doylestown, PA
Editor: The Editorium, Pipersville, PA
Manufacturing: Thompson-Shore, Dexter, MI

ZonePress
P.O. Box 1778, Doylestown, PA 18901

ISBN 0-9666302-0-3

Library of Congress catalog card number: 98-090656
Printed and bound in the United States of America

To Tom, a true champion

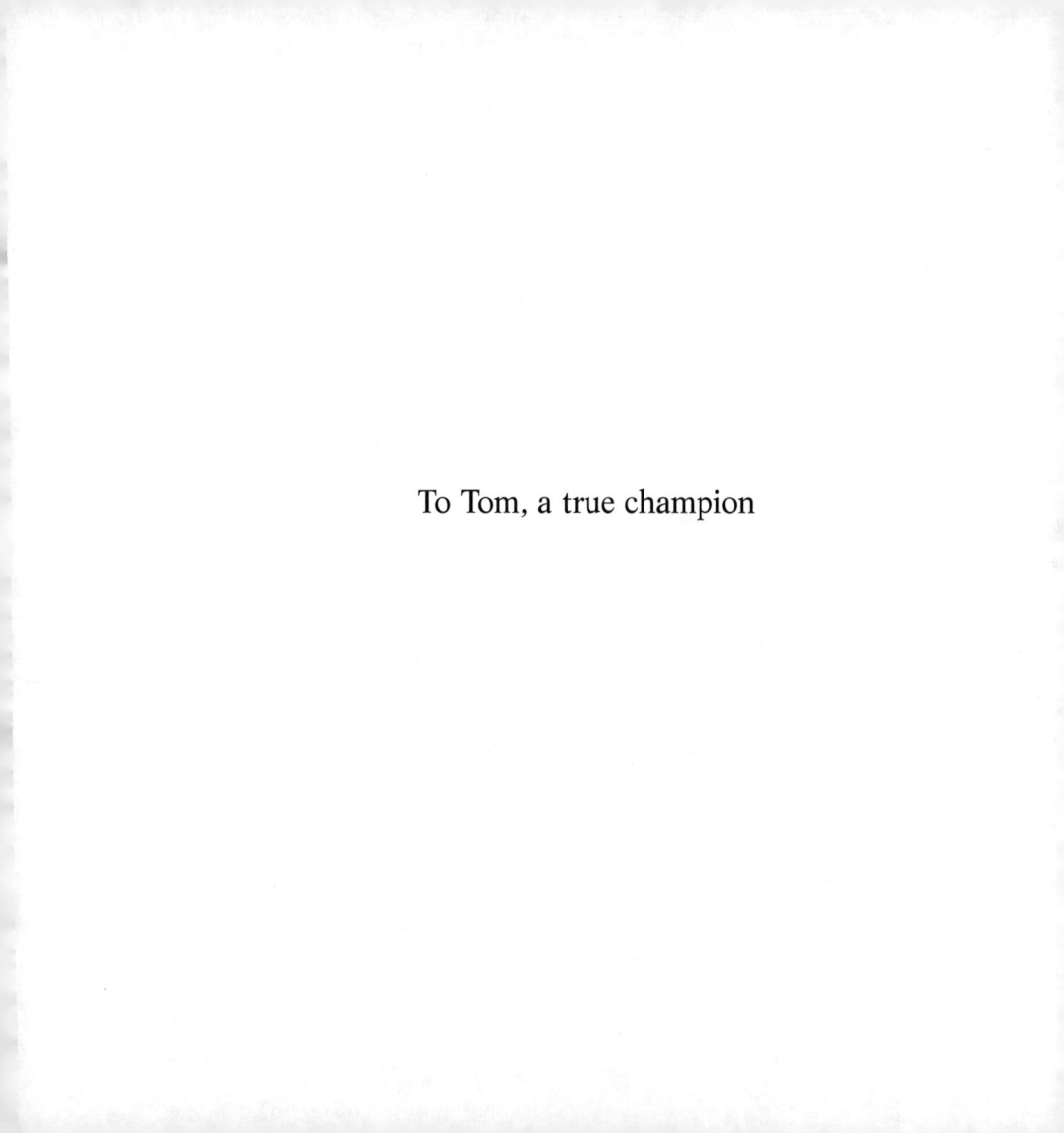

But...Who is Gymrat?

Gymrat is an authority on athletic development, and he is quickly becoming the sports philosopher of our time. His Rat-Chat is raising eyebrows. Gymrat publishes two question/answer columns, one for athletes and one for parents and coaches of young athletes. Both can be viewed at GymbagWisdom.com. Since making his home on the World Wide Web, the world has become his new gymnasium. Now everyone can benefit from his wisdom.

Attention!
As always, consult a physician before engaging in any exercise program.

CONTENTS

PREFACE i
INTRODUCTION iii

Physical Rat-Chat Advice

SWIFTER ON YOUR FEET

#1	The Best Training Device	3
#2	Sports-Specific Runs	5
#3	Pick' em Up, Put' em Down	. .6
#4	Somersaults	8
#5	Bounce Around	9
#6	Ballet Lessons?	10

STRENGTH AND POWER

#7	My "Quick Jump" Test	12
#8	Squat On One Leg	14
#9	Girls, Add Strength	16
#10	The Missing Link	18
#11	Baby Steps	19
#12	Add Some Springs	20
#13	More Than A Warm-Up	21

THE NEED FOR SPEED

#14	Run Quietly	24
#15	The Unexpected Benefit Of Flexibility	26
#16	Downhill Running	27

FUEL FOR ATHLETES

#17	Eat To Compete	30
#18	The Most Important Nutrient	32
#19	What About Vitamins?	33

SURE HANDS

#20	While Studying?	35
#21	One-Handed Catch	37

SMART-TRAINING METHODS

#22	Seeing Is Believing	39
#23	Zero In	40
#24	Instant Pancakes	41
#25	The K.I.S.S. Principle	42
#26	What The Elite All Have In Common	43

#	Title	Page
#27	Like A Sand Pile	44
#28	The Balance Beam	45
#29	The Key To Success	47
#30	Cross-Playing	48
#31	Learn To Prevent Them	49

Mental And Emotional Rat-Chat Advice

MENTAL GYMNASTICS

#	Title	Page
#32	My "Sign Of A Good Athletic Mind" Quiz	53
#33	Enter The Zone	55
#34	Practice Tuning Out Distractions	56
#35	Another Arrow In Your Quiver	58
#36	Feel Your Muscles Twitching	59
#37	Headphones—A Time And A Place	60
#38	Mental Reruns	62
#39	Prepare For A Perfect Practice	63

WINNING APPROACH

#	Title	Page
#40	It Takes Steel To Sharpen Steel	65
#41	A Natural Athlete	66
#42	"Paralysis Thru Analysis"	67
#43	Always Come To Compete	68
#44	Work Hard At Working Smart	70
#45	It's All About Confidence	71
#46	Sometimes You Can Try Too Hard	72
#47	G.A.M.E.R.	73
#48	No Sweat	74
#49	Even When You're Injured	75

WINNING WAYS

#	Title	Page
#50	The Reset Generation	77
#51	Like An Iditarod Sled Dog	78
#52	The "Sixth Sense"	79
#53	Yo-Yo	80
#54	They Paid Their Dues	82
#55	The Mark Of A Champion	83
#56	Think Feedback, Not Setback	84

#	Title	Page
#57	Learn To End Up In First	85
#58	F.I.R.S.T.	86
#59	Play To Win	87
#60	Quality Practice	88
#61	Winning Is A Mind-set	89
#62	Second Best Is For The Rest	90
#63	The Big Mistakes	91
#64	Success Is Earned	92
#65	Program Yourself	93

MOTIVATION

#	Title	Page
#66	The Opportunity Of Summer	94
#67	L.O.S.E.R.	96
#68	No Luck About It	97
#69	You Have To Risk	98
#70	"Can't" Never Achieved Anything	99
#71	Don't Label Yourself	100
#72	Pre-Game Pep "Self" Talk	101
#73	They're Out There	102
#74	You May Be A Late Bloomer	103
#75	It Takes Courage	104
#76	It's Worse Than Losing	105
#77	Keep The Streak Going	106
#78	Could Of—Should Of	107

IN CONTROL

#	Title	Page
#79	G.U.T.S.	109
#80	A Seasoned Veteran	110
#81	Pressure Can Be A Good Thing	111
#82	The Magic Is In The Air	112
#83	Be The Calm That Settles The Sea	114
#84	Sports Rituals	115
#85	The Cream Rises To The Top	116
#86	Cage The Rage	117

THE OLD FASHION WAY

#87	Be A Grizzly	119
#88	To Make Real Progress	120
#89	Self-Pride	121
#90	Push Yourself	122
#91	Adversity Will Make You Stronger	123
#92	No Fatigue Pain, No Gain	124

CREATING THE WILL

#93	The "Eye Of The Tiger"	126
#94	Stoking The Fire	128
#95	Unravel The Mystery	129
#96	The Most Common Regret	130

SUPPORT SYSTEMS

#97	Be Coachable	132
#98	Pack Of Wolves	133
#99	Give Thanks	134
#100	Building Team Spirit	135

LOCKER ROOM WRAP-UP

#101	May The Force Be With You	138
#102	Keep Your Head Up	140
#103	The Big Lie	141
#104	Feel Like A Champion	142
#105	The Golden Sports Rule	143
#106	It's Not The Size Of The Trophy	144

PREFACE

What is your AQ? No, not your Intelligent Quotient, but your *Athletic Quotient*? Answer this question to see if you have the natural desire to be an athlete:

Your favorite sport is on television, but the sun is out and the opportunity for you to play the same sport presents itself. Do you lace them up or is it couch city?

Turn the page to see how you scored...

If you were lacing them up before you even finished reading the first part, you have a high AQ.

To become a better athlete, you must have a desire to be more of a doer than a watcher.

INTRODUCTION

Unlike other books that focus only on developing one aspect of the athlete, this book provides lessons for becoming a complete athlete. Each page in this book presents a different lesson, arranged in no particular order.

While the big opportunity is for the young maturing athlete, it's not too late for the college, elite, or even the millions of recreational athletes who want to take their game to a new level. They, too, can improve athletically, especially mentally and emotionally.

As you pass through adolescence, you are presented with windows of opportunity for developing your athletic ability. It's important that you engage in proper training techniques because once you pass through these windows, there's no going back. Seize the opportunity! Achieving the peak of your potential someday depends on the foundation of athletic ability (physically and mentally) you develop when you're young.

But to tap into what's hidden in your genes, you must train smart. Did you know that just by improving your technique, you'll be able to run faster? Just like a car, if you become more efficient, you won't need a bigger engine to go faster. And did you know that visualization will help you perform at your best in the clutch, or that mental imagery will help improve your physical skills?

This book will also motivate and inspire you. It will help you understand what it takes to reach your goals, to fulfill your dreams. After you read this book, keep it handy. Any time you get a few moments, re-read a lesson or two. Some lessons can be applied right away, but many will need reviewing to sink in.

Physical Rat-Chat Advice

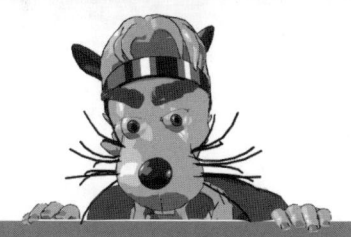

SWIFTER ON YOUR FEET

#1 The Best Training Device
#2 Sports-Specific Runs
#3 Pick' em Up, Put' em Down
#4 Somersaults
#5 Bounce Around
#6 Ballet Lessons?

#1 The Best Training Device

Even with today's technology, the jump rope is still the best device for developing your athletic ability—it can do wonders for foot speed, agility, quickness, and coordination. All it takes is ten minutes a day.

No aspiring athlete should be without a jump rope. It's the second most important thing that goes into your gym bag (this book is first, of course). Sometimes the simplest things in life have the greatest value.

SWIFTER ON YOUR FEET

Once you get the hang of skipping rope, mix up your patterns. Jump rope backwards, crisscross your hands, alternate jumping from one foot to the other. Be creative with the rope; challenge your feet. As your jump roping skills improve, you will notice yourself, in general, becoming swifter and lighter on your feet. Keep the rope moving, and you'll soon become a better athlete.

#2 Sports-Specific Runs

Out on your training runs, you can become a better athlete. How? Simply mix up your running style. Rather than spending the entire time running straight ahead, do some skipping, hopping, cross-overs, backward running, and side to side shuffling. Work hard. It's a great way, and a great time to develop your foot speed, agility, and your overall athletic coordination. After the first ten minutes of your run, switch every fifty yards to a different style until your run is over. If your sport requires you to do more than straight ahead running, you need to incorporate that type of running into your training runs.

SWIFTER ON YOUR FEET

#3 Pick' em Up, Put' em Down

The Dot drill: a great way to improve your agility and foot quickness. Mark these spots on the floor with tape. Approximately two feet apart.

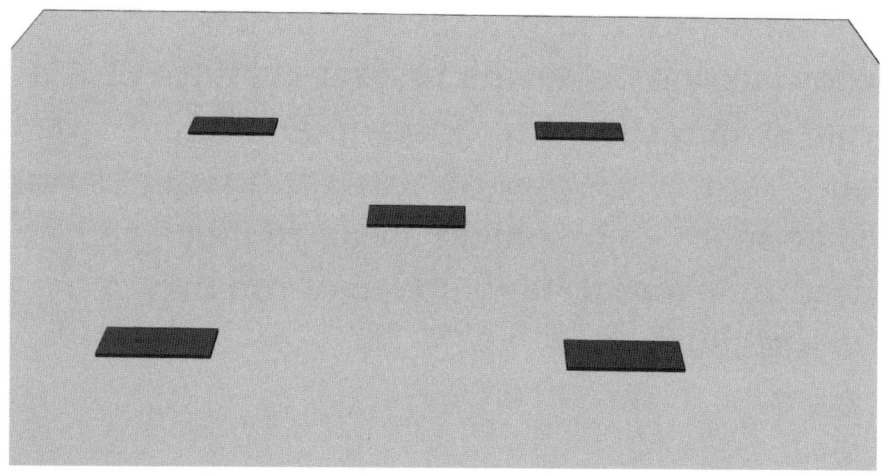

The object is to move from one dot to the other as quickly as possible. Create your own patterns. Choose two patterns per workout. For each pattern, do a set with both feet together and then a set with each foot separately. Practice until you get the hang of a pattern and then start the clock. Move around the pattern as fast as you can for fifteen seconds. Strive to break your previous record for each pattern. Since the object is to move as quickly as possible, make sure you are well rested between sets. Perform at least three times a week for three months.

#4 Somersaults

Somersaults aren't just for kids. Great athletes of all sports include forward and backward rolls into their conditioning programs. And not just for fun either. They are a great way to develop overall body control and coordination. Somersaults help athletes develop kinesthetic awareness. In other words, they help them improve their athletic ability, and they also teach athletes how to fall safely (tuck and roll). Start out performing them from the knees, then standing, and then progress to running and rolling.

#5 Bounce Around

A mini-trampoline can help you improve your lower body strength and endurance. At the same time it can help you develop better balance, coordination, and overall body control. Bounce around. Master all kinds of moves on the tramp—develop a strong sense of movement. The more creative you are on the mini-tramp, the more athletic ability you will develop.

SWIFTER ON YOUR FEET

#6 Ballet Lessons?

Many great athletes supplement their training and conditioning programs with ballet lessons—and for good reason. Learning how to float around the ballet floor is one of the best ways to improve your athletic ability for sports. Ballet will enhance your coordination, body control, and help you become more graceful and lighter on your feet. Ballet dancers and athletes may be a world apart culturally, but when it comes to physical abilities, they're close in nature.

STRENGTH AND POWER

#7 My "Quick Jump" Test
#8 Squat On One Leg
#9 Girls, Add Strength
#10 The Missing Link
#11 Baby Steps
#12 Add Some Springs
#13 More Than A Warm-Up

STRENGTH AND POWER

#7 My "Quick Jump" Test

If you want to improve your jumping ability use the "quick jump" test as an exercise—it will give you some serious "hops." Here is how the "quick jump" test works. First, find your maximal vertical jump and divide that number by two (that is called your predetermined number). Then stand flat-footed against a wall or under the basket with an arm extended as high as possible. Take the predetermined number and measure upward from your extended fingertip and mark that spot on the wall or backboard.

The object is to see how many times you can jump up and touch that spot in ten seconds. As you are able to jump up to that spot more times in ten seconds, you'll become a quicker and tireless jumper—you'll be ready for today's style of game. Build up to four sets of the quick jump test, three times a week. Make sure you warm up first and build gradually before you give it your all every set, every workout. Do the program for at least three months and gain some real "ups."

STRENGTH AND POWER

#8 Squat On One Leg

One-legged squats are a great and safe way to develop your lower body strength and improve your balance at the same time. Here's how: Stand on one leg with arms out to the side. While keeping the free leg extended out in front, squat down slightly. Pause a moment and then rise back up. As you get stronger and your balance improves, squat lower on each repetition. Your goal is to eventually squat down until the thigh you're squatting with is parallel to the floor and no lower.

Do three sets of your maximum, three times a week. To experience the best results from this program, continue for at least six months.

GYMBAG WISDOM - 106 Ways To Become A Better Athlete

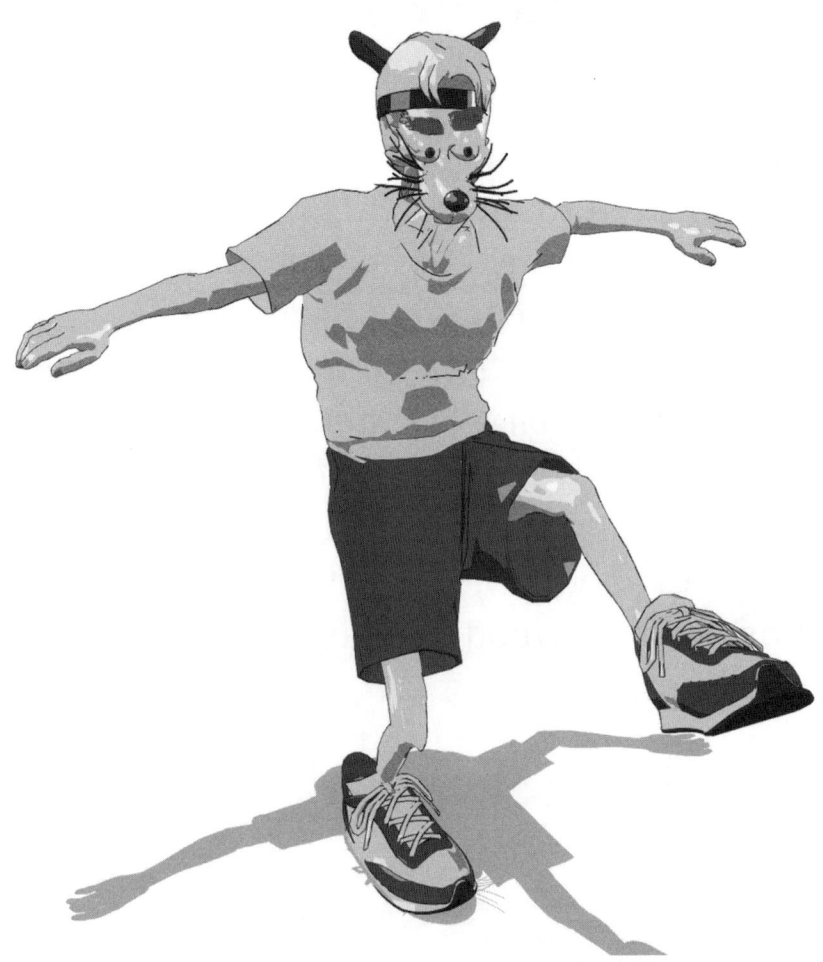

STRENGTH AND POWER

#9 Girls, Add Strength

Since girls are taking sports as seriously as boys, they need to increase their strength. Boys usually come from a more physically active background. Girls enter sports less well-prepared physically. They're further away from their strength potential than boys, which means that girls actually have more to gain from strength training. Stay away from the weights until you're about 14, or 15, but long before that hammer down on push-ups, shoulder dips, and pull-ups.

Girls' performance will improve over the years, and greater strength will be the main reason. Girls will get stronger and catch up to their strength potential at younger ages. This will allow them to pass through their athletic development years with stronger bodies. As a result, they will mature into better athletes.

STRENGTH AND POWER

#10 The Missing Link

The mid-body is an important link. Every athletic movement in sports revolves around the mid-body, yet it's normally the most under-trained body part of an athlete. When it comes to strength and conditioning, athletes tend to focus most of their time and energy developing their upper and lower body while neglecting their low back and abdominal muscles. Like a chain, an athlete's body is only as strong as its weakest link. Make sure you're doing at least fifteen minutes of trunk exercises three times a week. Examples: sit-ups (rotate elbow to opposite knee), crunches, leg lifts.

#11 Baby Steps

Be careful not to do too much too soon. When it comes to conditioning, increase the intensity gradually. If you rush to the high intensity stuff too quickly, your body will break down and you'll end up regressing rather than progressing. Whether it's a running program or a strength and conditioning program, adding five percent a week is an ideal progression.

STRENGTH AND POWER

#12 Add Some Springs

Plyometrics are high intensity bounding exercises used for enhancing power. They put spring into your legs. They put bounce into your stride. Plyometrics help you run faster and jump higher. But since they're very demanding on the body, you'll need to develop a strong base of conditioning before they can be safely and effectively added to your workout program. When you've trained properly and worked up to plyometrics, they will help you become a better athlete.

#13 More Than A Warm-Up

Push-ups, pull-ups, and shoulder dips are more than just warm-up exercises. Many of today's best athletes use them as their main strength and conditioning exercises. These exercises work the major muscle groups of the upper body, and if the body is held as stiff as an ironing board when performing push-ups, it's a great way to develop low back and abdominal strength. But you really have to push yourself in order to receive maximum benefits from these exercises. Keep in mind that until you can adequately lift your own body weight, you won't need free weights to get stronger.

STRENGTH AND POWER

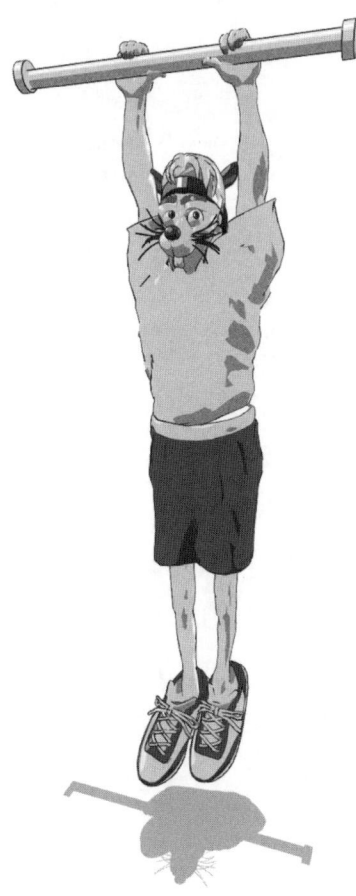

THE NEED FOR SPEED

#14 Run Quietly
#15 The Unexpected Benefit Of Flexibility
#16 Downhill Running

THE NEED FOR SPEED

#14 Run Quietly

If you simply improve your running technique, you'll be able to run faster. A great way to automatically improve your technique is to practice running quietly. When you develop the skill of setting your feet down softly, your entire running gait becomes more efficient. A more efficient runner is a faster runner. When you begin the practice of running quietly, start out slowly and build gradually. Since you'll be using running muscles a new way, the proper way, initially it can be a bit taxing on your lower legs.

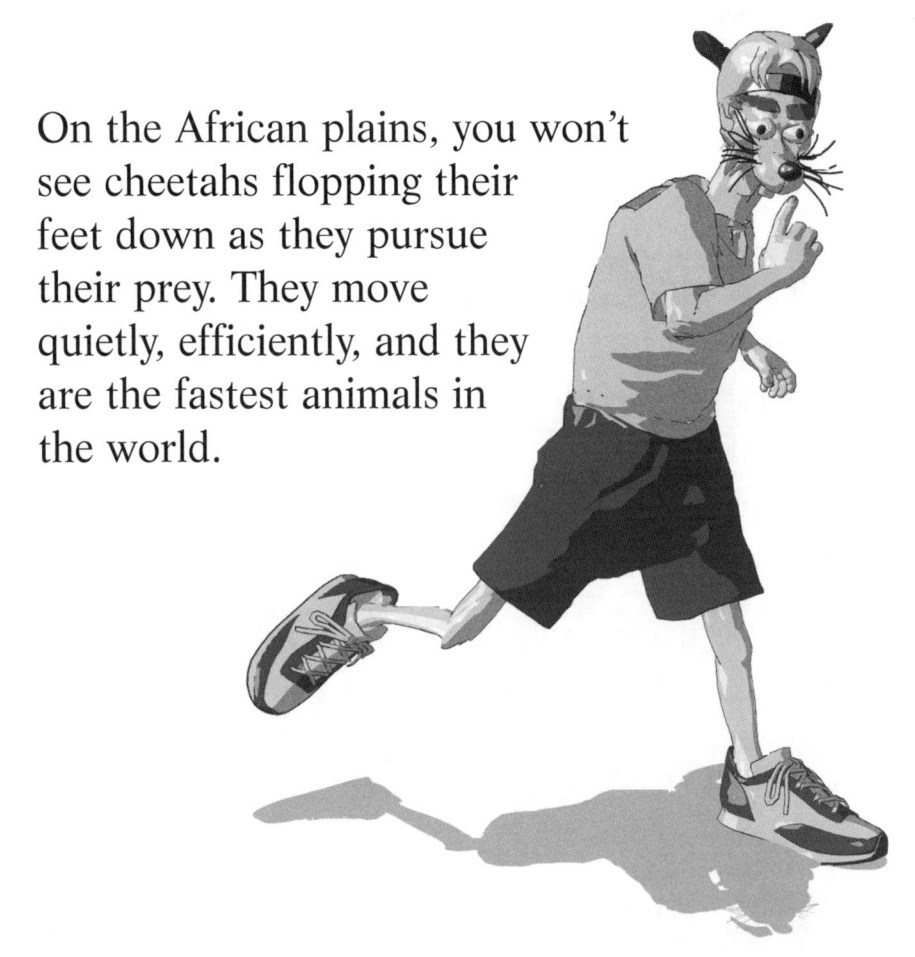

On the African plains, you won't see cheetahs flopping their feet down as they pursue their prey. They move quietly, efficiently, and they are the fastest animals in the world.

THE NEED FOR SPEED

#15 The Unexpected Benefit Of Flexibility

Stretch yourself to new limits. Did you know that you can improve your speed simply by improving your lower body flexibility? Tight muscles limit your range of motion. Increasing your flexibility increases your stride length. With a longer stride, you will cover more ground in less time and with less energy. You will be able to run faster simply by becoming more flexible.

Work on limbering up the following four: (1) hamstrings (2) hips (3) calves (4) quadriceps.

#16 Downhill Running

Running downhill can help you improve your speed on flat terrain. Downhill running opens up your stride and develops the type of strength that prevents one from "sinking" on each step. The less your legs "give" on impact, the more spring they will have when they uncoil and push off.

After you have developed a solid base of conditioning from running on flat terrain and inclines, it's time to find a gradual decline. The rule of thumb: If the decline forces you to change your gait, or makes you feel like your applying the brakes so not to fall over forward, the hill is too steep.

THE NEED FOR SPEED

When you begin your workout, warm up with a fifteen minute run on flat terrain followed by a ten minute stretching session. Your workout should include two sets each of 50 meters, 100 meters and 200 hundred meters. After each set jog back up. In the beginning weeks give about 80 percent in every set, and then reach for ninety and one hundred percent effort in the last weeks of your program (six to eight weeks total). Perform no more than twice a week, and have at least three days rest in between each workout. On the other days, continue your base training by running on flat terrain.

FUEL FOR ATHLETES

#17 Eat To Compete
#18 The Most Important Nutrient
#19 What About Vitamins?

FUEL FOR ATHLETES

#17 Eat To Compete

Eat to compete. If a piece of paper and a piece of charcoal are set on fire at the same time, which of the two burns up quicker? It's a no-brainer. The paper would go up in a blaze and quickly burn out, and the charcoal would burn long and slow. Refined sugars, such as candy bars and cookies, are like the paper. In the beginning they give you a burst of energy, but then they quickly leave you depleted. Snacks such as pretzels, fruits, veggies, and whole-wheat breads are like the charcoal; they burn slowly and sustain you the entire game.

GYMBAG WISDOM - 106 Ways To Become A Better Athlete

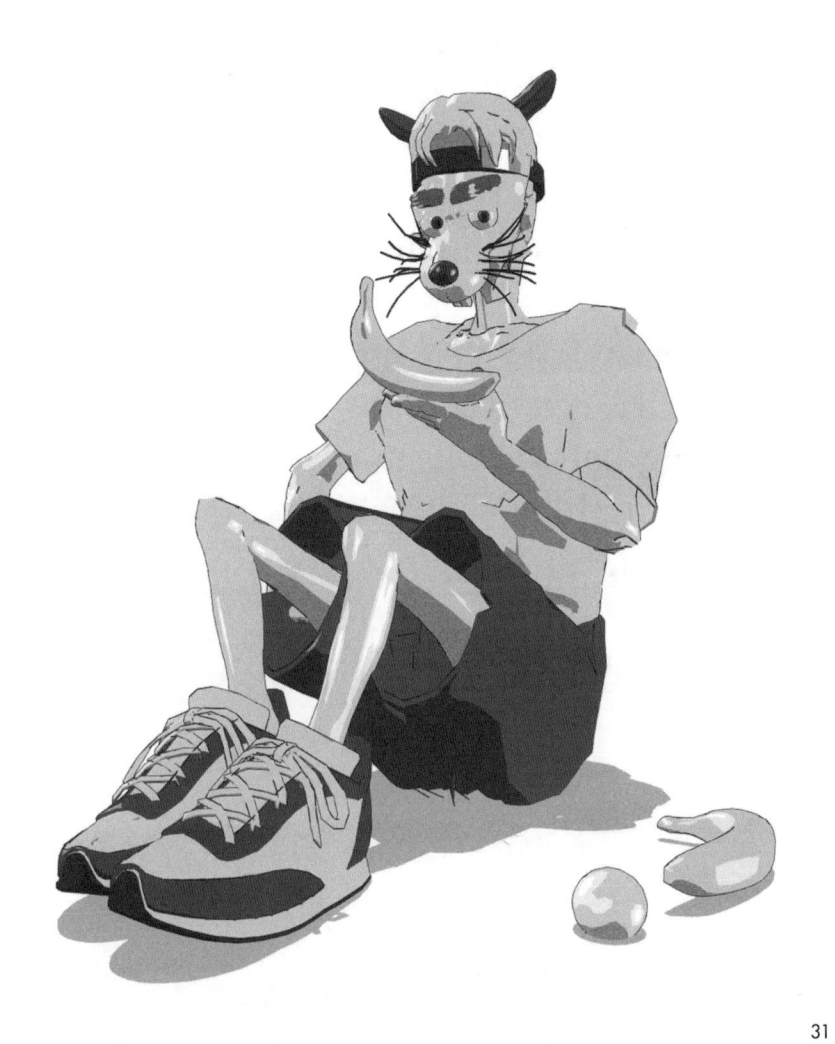

FUEL FOR ATHLETES

#18 The Most Important Nutrient

Sports drinks are popular, but you don't always need them when you become thirsty. In fact, only if you're engaged in continuous, strenuous exercise can they make a difference in your performance. Your body will require water long before it'll need sport drinks. Water is an athlete's most important nutrient. But you'll never hear that from the companies that sell sport drinks. Listen to the experts, not the commercials.

#19 What About Vitamins?

Do athletes need vitamin supplements? Like anybody else, only if they're not eating healthy everyday. Athletes who work out hard, however, need more calories than the average person. If the extra food they consume is nutritious, they will get all the vitamins their bodies will require. Your body can only use so many vitamins at one time. It's called the water-bucket theory; you can pour only so much water in a bucket before it overflows. Be careful not to fall into the trap of taking vitamins to make up for a poor diet, or as a last ditch effort to improve your stamina.

SURE HANDS

#20 While Studying?
#21 One-Handed Catch

#20 While Studying?

Studying is a great time to develop better hands. When it's time for a break, practice juggling. It's a fun activity that enhances your hand-eye coordination and improves your focus skills. The catching skills you develop from juggling will carry over and help you in your sport. In return, juggling during study breaks clears your mind. When you return to the books, your mind will be more relaxed and better able to understand and comprehend what you were working on.

SURE HANDS

Sorry, hand-eye coordination cannot be developed from playing video games. Hand-eye coordination is developed only from activities that require you to move your hand toward and then to grasp what your eyes are converging on. The only physical coordination development going on when playing video games is your thumb pushing a button.

#21 One-Handed Catch

A great way to develop better hands is to practice playing catch with a football one-handed. Toss the ball up into the air on your own, or play catch with a partner. As you improve, toss the ball farther or harder. Because a football has such an oblong shape, you have to focus intently and grasp delicately in order to make a one-handed catch. As your one-handed catching ability improves with a football, catching anything with two hands will become easier.

SMART-TRAINING METHODS

#22 Seeing Is Believing
#23 Zero In
#24 Instant Pancakes
#25 The K.I.S.S. Principle
#26 What The Elite All Have In Common
#27 Like A Sand Pile
#28 The Balance Beam
#29 The Key To Success
#30 Cross-Playing
#31 Learn To Prevent Them

#22 Seeing Is Believing

In addition to using your video camera for capturing your great game performances, use it to help you improve. The video camera is one of the best training aids for athletes. A coach can tell you over and over, but until you see yourself on film, you may never understand what you're doing wrong. Seeing is believing. There's nothing like visual feedback to open your eyes to what you're doing incorrectly or correctly. Tape yourself at least once a week. Study the details, and watch yourself improve.

SMART-TRAINING METHODS

#23 Zero In

Take dead aim. When you're about to shoot a free throw, attempt a crucial putt, or do anything that requires precise accuracy, don't just look at your target—see it. Stare at it intently until you have the details in sight. Give your eyes the time to adjust and focus like binoculars. When you hone in and study the details of your target, your eyes will be better able to register the range in your brain. If you give your target just a glance, you don't stand much of a chance.

#24 Instant Pancakes

Shape yourself into a player—don't try to play yourself into shape. You can't adequately prepare for the season in a couple of weeks. You can't expect to be much better if you don't work hard the entire off-season. It takes months, not weeks, to significantly improve your skills and to adequately condition for any sport. You can just add water and get instant pancakes but there's no such thing as developing instant athletes.

SMART-TRAINING METHODS

#25 The K.I.S.S. Principle

THE K.I.S.S. PRINCIPLE
(Keep It Sport Specific)

It's important to incorporate exercises into your training program that mirror the type of movements required in your sport. For example, since a throwing motion, a tennis swing, a slap shot, or any skill that requires your mid-body to twist and contract at the same time you execute, you should do sit-ups with a twist. Alternate elbow to opposite knee. This will develop the mid-body muscles in the way they assist you in those skills. Keep your training specific to your sport and you'll benefit more from your workouts.

#26 What The Elite All Have In Common

Master the fundamentals. With any activity, great fundamentals are what the elite all have in common. Never take them too lightly. The secret to excelling at sports, school, music, dance, or any skill activity, is to excel at the fundamentals first. When you have a flare for the basics, the difficult skills are easier to develop.

SMART-TRAINING METHODS

#27 Like A Sand Pile

Develop a solid foundation. When it comes to strength and conditioning programs, it's essential that you build a solid base of conditioning before engaging in high intensity exercises such as speed work and plyometrics. Build slowly and build thoroughly; your health and your potential are at stake. Like a sand pile, the size of your foundation determines how high you'll eventually peak.

#28 The Balance Beam

A great way to improve your balance for sports is to practice sport skills on a balance beam. You don't need a traditional balance beam found in a gym; simply lay a two-by-four on the ground. Perform any skill: swing a bat, a golf club, a tennis racket, or toss up a ball and catch it. Practicing sport skills on a balance beam will give you a finely tuned sense of balance.

SMART-TRAINING METHODS

Whatever skill you do on the beam, perform in slow motion first. As your balance improves, increase your speed. And when you are ready for the ultimate challenge, try the activity you're doing with your eyes closed. Work on the beam and you'll put balance into your game.

#29 The Key To Success

Even with all the great sports equipment available today, a combination of practice, hard work, and guts is still what separates the winners from the losers. Good equipment is important but you can't buy success. Keep in mind that it isn't the expensive machinery that brings out your best, but the condition of the machine using the equipment.

SMART-TRAINING METHODS

#30 Cross-Playing

To become a better athlete, play other sports. The athletic ability developed from one sport will carry over and help you excel in other sports. For example, the agility developed in soccer will help in tennis. Wrestlers make good football players because they understand leverage. Skating helps one to ski because the athletic principles of transferring weight are the same. Cross-playing helps one become an all-around better athlete. Many great athletes have said that the coordination and mental toughness they developed from other sports helped them to excel in the one they do best.

#31 Learn To Prevent Them

Ankle sprains are the number one time-loss sports injury. To help prevent them, stretch ankles just as you would your muscles before activity. Here's how: While standing, roll one ankle over to the outside and for fifteen seconds gradually push down. Repeat with other. Now if the ankle twists or rolls over while playing it will tend to "give" more before an injury takes place. One of the easiest ways to become a better athlete is to stay injury free.

SMART-TRAINING METHODS

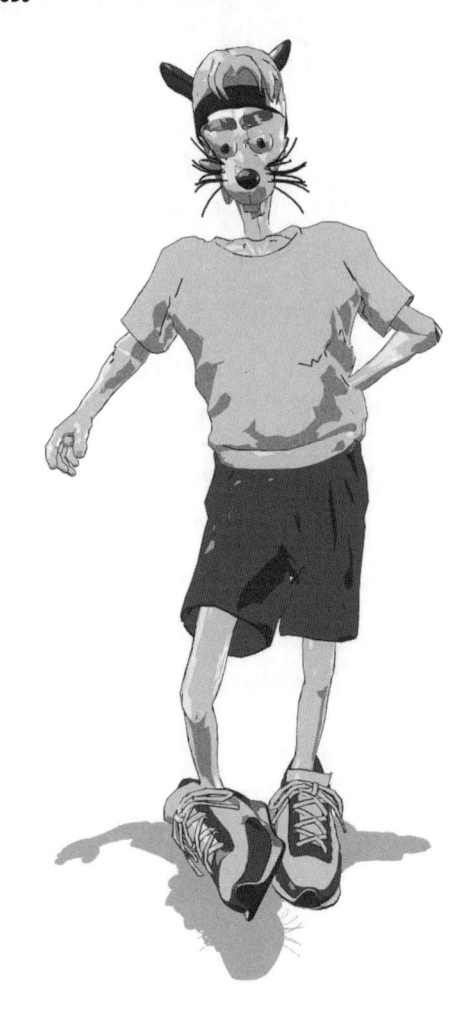

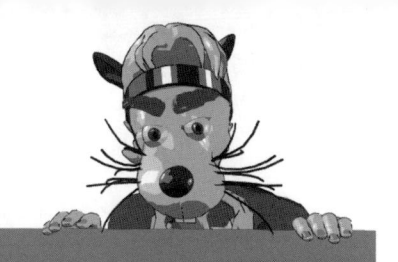

Mental And Emotional Rat-Chat Advice

MENTAL GYMNASTICS

#32 My "Sign Of A Good Athletic Mind" Quiz
#33 Enter The Zone
#34 Practice Tuning Out Distractions
#35 Another Arrow In Your Quiver
#36 Feel Your Muscles Twitching
#37 Headphones—A Time And A Place
#38 Mental Reruns
#39 Prepare For A Perfect Practice

#32 My "Sign Of A Good Athletic Mind" Quiz

Try the "Sign of a good athletic mind" quiz.

Sit down, close your eyes, and focus only on your breathing. The trick is to see if you can count ten breaths in a row without being distracted. Only think of your breathing and nothing else. Stop and take the quiz now and then read on to the next page.

The scoring is simple. If you fell short of ten breaths in a row before being distracted, it's time to get serious about working on your mental toughness. If you made it all the way to ten, you still failed. Why? Because how can you focus "only" on your breathing and still be able to count your breaths?

To pass the quiz with flying colors your answer had to be something like, "I don't know how many breaths I took before being distracted, but it seemed like a lot." The purpose of this trick quiz is to give you an idea of the awareness it takes to play "in the zone."

#33 Enter The Zone

Reaching the "zone" is the pinnacle of sports. Once experienced, it's what every athlete strives for the rest of his playing days. Playing "in the zone" is the ultimate lure of sports. It is a special time when your mind quiets and your senses take over. It's when everything you can do in practice flows out in a game like it was second nature. Stay focused on the "now" long enough and everything will become easy and effortless—everything will begin to click. Suddenly, it will feel as if you were switched to automatic pilot—you'll have entered the "zone."

MENTAL GYMNASTICS

#34 Practice Tuning Out Distractions

In order to improve your focus skills, you need to learn how to tune out distractions. Here's a great drill. Take out a book that you need to read for school and crank the music. For thirty seconds, mentally tune out the music and focus only on reading. Then switch and for thirty seconds listen to the music as intently as you read. Change back and forth ten times. Perform once a day. Work hard at staying focused, and in a few weeks your concentration will improve dramatically. Whether it's in sports or in the classroom, possessing strong focus skills will take you to the next level.

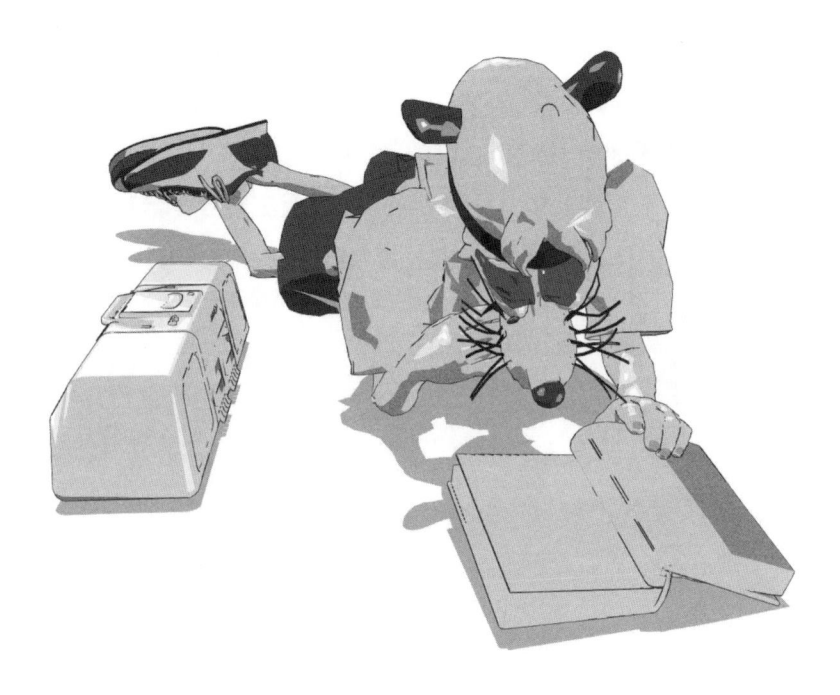

GYMBAG WISDOM—106 Ways To Become A Better Athlete

MENTAL GYMNASTICS

#35 Another Arrow In Your Quiver

Before a game or even a practice, take a few moments to picture yourself performing at your best. If you take the time and energy to mentally rehearse, you can gain an edge before the whistle even blows. Don't just show up and hope to do your best, first visualize what you need to do to be your best. Visualization is another weapon for competition. It's another arrow in your quiver.

#36 Feel Your Muscles Twitching

When you're learning a new skill or trying to improve on an existing one, take time to visualize it first. Run it through your mind several times before attempting it for real. First in slow motion to get the perfect technique, then see yourself executing it perfectly at regular speed. Concentrate so hard you can feel your muscles twitching as you run the image through your mind. When you go to practice the real thing, don't think about it—just do it. Allow the muscle memory that you developed from visualization to take over.

MENTAL GYMNASTICS

#37 Headphones—A Time And A Place

When you head out to run, leave the headphones behind. To get the most out of your runs, you must work at staying focused on your technique, breathing, and rhythm. Even on your training runs, learn to keep your mind still, centered, and on the task at hand. To develop a strong athletic mind, you need to maintain the same mind-set in training as you do in games. Successful athletes use their training runs to develop mental toughness as well as stamina.

Listening to headphones can help you stay relaxed before competition, but when it's time to work out they become a distraction. Keep in mind you can't use music to motivate you in a game when things get tough, so don't try to use it to get you through a tough workout.

MENTAL GYMNASTICS

#38 Mental Reruns

Take the time and energy for mental reruns. Soon after the game ends, replay moments in your mind. Review and study what you did right or what you did wrong. Relive the moment while it's still fresh in your mind. If you had a great performance, rerun it, reinforce it twenty times. If you had a bad game, mentally correct your mistakes twenty times. Just as rewriting your notes immediately after a class can help you understand the lesson, replaying a game in your head soon after it was played can do the same.

#39 Prepare For A Perfect Practice

After the bell goes off and school is out for the day, start day dreaming about the energy you'll need for a great practice. As you walk back to your locker and chat with friends, start getting pumped. Get into the game frame of mind right from the school-ending bell and your practice will get off to a bang. Mentally preparing for a perfect practice will increase your chances of practicing perfectly.

WINNING APPROACH

#40 It Takes Steel To Sharpen Steel
#41 A Natural Athlete
#42 "Paralysis Thru Analysis"
#43 Always Come To Compete
#44 Work Hard At Working Smart
#45 It's All About Confidence
#46 Sometimes You Can Try Too Hard
#47 G.A.M.E.R.
#48 No Sweat
#49 Even When You're Injured

#40 It Takes Steel To Sharpen Steel

To get better at your sport you need a challenge. Tough competition is what sharpens your skills, not the easy wins. Don't duck a better opponent because you might lose. Get up for the challenge. Look at tough competition as an invitation to get better. To sharpen your skills, you need something that can match your strength. It takes steel to sharpen steel.

WINNING APPROACH

#41 A Natural Athlete

Everybody starts out as a natural athlete in childhood, but very few continue to be one as they grow up. Somewhere along the way, most lose the gift. A child's approach to play is natural—free of self-concept, free of mental resistance, and absent of emotional barriers and fears. Approach sports as you did when you were a child, and you will rediscover the natural athlete that lies within us all.

#42 "Paralysis Thru Analysis"

The sure way to fall into a slump, or to stay in a slump, is to over-analyze. Athletes often think themselves into a frenzy. They get their minds so preoccupied with over-analyzing, and giving themselves instruction, they freeze up when it's time to perform. They develop "paralysis thru analysis." In sports, there is a time to think and a time to do. When it's time to do, suppress the thinker and activate the doer. A great baseball player once said, "You can't think and hit a baseball at the same time."

WINNING APPROACH

#43 Always Come To Compete

Become a competitor. Any time you lace them up, put the game face on. Even in practice, never drop your guard. Rise to the occasion anytime someone challenges your game. Protect your domain. Allow your natural instincts to take over and your competitive juices to flow. Make it a pride thing—always come to compete. Champions are forged in the fire of competition.

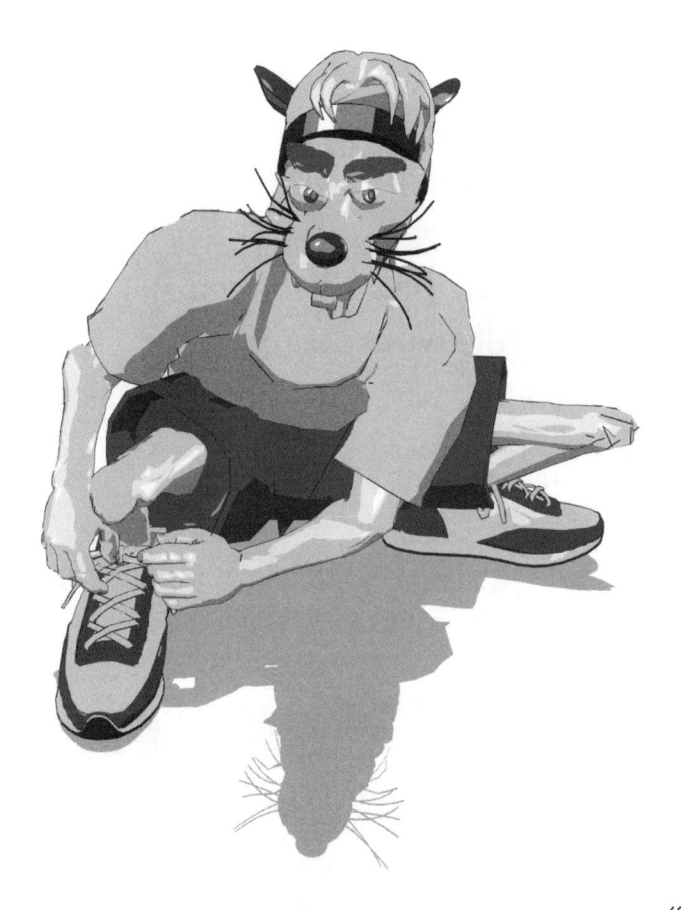

GYMBAG WISDOM—106 Ways To Become A Better Athlete

WINNING APPROACH

#44 Work Hard At Working Smart

Work smarter, not just harder. When it comes time to take your game, or any activity to a new high, improve your efficiency before you put in the extra hard work. Find out the smartest way of getting it done before you bear down. Strain your brain before you begin to strain your body. Work hard at working smart and you'll achieve more.

#45 It's All About Confidence

The secret to gaining confidence in sports is preparation. Sit down with your coach and plan each practice in the off-season with an attainable goal in mind, then work that plan. Prepare your practices so you can succeed one step at a time. Success breeds success. With hard work comes competence, and with competence comes confidence.

WINNING APPROACH

#46 Sometimes You Can Try Too Hard

You never can work too hard, but sometimes you can try too hard. When you practice something over and over and just can't seem to make progress, back off for awhile. Take some time to clear your mind. Learning skills cannot be forced. After taking a short break, go at it again. As with training a dog, you'll make more progress if your training sessions are shorter but more frequent.

#47 G.A.M.E.R.

Are you a G.A.M.E.R? (Giving it your all, Alert and aggressive, Mentally composed, Emotionally charged, Ready to play.)

Gamers are battlers—they're at their best when it matters. Gamers are players who show up pumped for the big games, and don't let up until the show is over. Teammates rally around them. Coaches depend on them. Loaded with pride and filled with confidence, Gamers come to play.

WINNING APPROACH

#48 No Sweat

Even when you're not practicing, you still can get better at your sport. How? Simply visualize yourself practicing. When you get free time throughout the day, engage in mental practice. Mental rehearsal trains the neural pathways. It helps you develop muscle memory without even playing. All it takes is a few moments here and there. Professional and Olympic athletes take full advantage of mental imagery to enhance their skills. Don't pass up on an opportunity to get better without even breaking a sweat.

#49 Even When You're Injured

When you sustain an injury apply ice for twenty minutes. Remove the ice. Wait a few hours, and then ice again. Ice three times a day for the first three days. During those three days elevate the injured area while icing. Also during the daytime (not overnight) keep an elastic wrap on the injured area for compression. Do everything you can to keep the swelling down—the speed of your recovery depends on it. And when you're icing, use that time to mentally rehearse your athletic skills. Even when you're injured, you can get better at your sport.

WINNING WAYS

#50 The Reset Generation
#51 Like An Iditarod Sled Dog
#52 The "Sixth Sense"
#53 Yo-Yo
#54 They Paid Their Dues
#55 The Mark Of A Champion
#56 Think Feedback, Not Setback
#57 Learn To End Up In First
#58 F.I.R.S.T.
#59 Play To Win
#60 Quality Practice
#61 Winning Is A Mind-set
#62 Second Best Is For The Rest
#63 The Big Mistakes
#64 Success Is Earned
#65 Program Yourself

#50 The Reset Generation

"Hey coach! Two strikes…two outs…bottom of the seventh…we're down by five, can I just reset it? Heck, that's what I do when I fall too far behind in a video game." Are you part of the reset generation? Does the reset button make quitting easy for you? Quitting is a habit—it doesn't matter where you pick it up.

When you are behind, put your pride on the line. Time might run out on you, but never quit. Always expect to come back. Develop a bad attitude toward giving up. Even in obvious defeat, never accept it, go down a fighter. This attitude will eventually turn you into a winner. Keep in mind, the more you quit, the easier quitting gets.

WINNING WAYS

#51 Like An Iditarod Sled Dog

Winners have learned to go full speed ahead all the time. No matter if it's practice or the real thing, they take it on with a full head of steam. They never have to give a second effort because they only play with continuous effort. Winners don't have a middle gear. They don't know what half speed is all about. Like an Iditarod sled dog, winners only know one speed—flat out.

#52 The "Sixth Sense"

Develop a winning instinct. When you have the lead late in the game, don't let your mind drift—don't start patting yourself on the back prematurely. Always expect one more big effort from your opponent that can steal the game from under your nose. Keep the intensity one step above your opponent's at all times. Stay in control of the momentum until the final whistle blows. Never give your opponent the feeling that he can recover. Develop a sixth sense for winning.

WINNING WAYS

#53 Yo-Yo

Do you find yourself performing like a yo-yo? Do you find yourself playing up or down to your opponent's level? If so, it's time for you to take control. It's time for you to show up for every game mentally ready to control the pace. In order to become a consistent winner, you must first learn to play with consistent intensity. Never allow your opponent to control you like a yo-yo on a string. Develop the mental stability to always play up to your athletic ability.

GYMBAG WISDOM—106 Ways To Become A Better Athlete

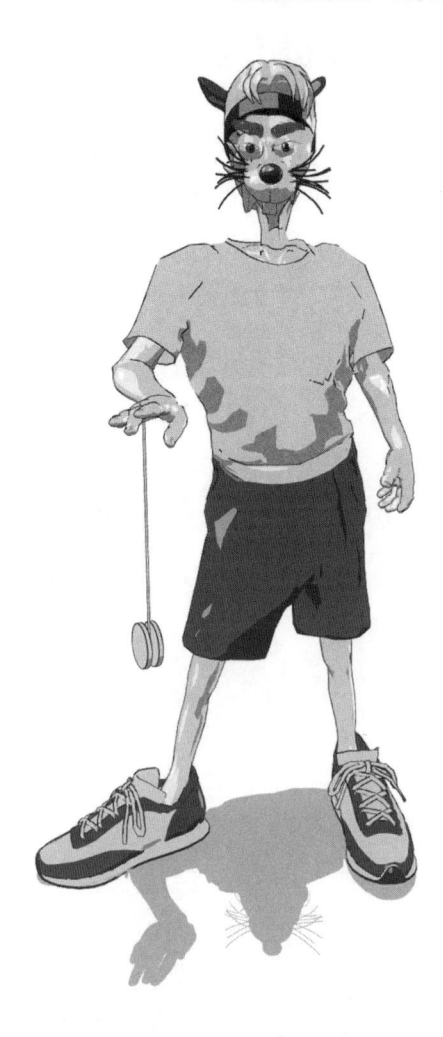

WINNING WAYS

#54 They Paid Their Dues

Champions are developed in the off-season. All the hours of practice, all the hard work, and all the sacrifices—these things will not be forgotten. When the season rolls around and crunch time nears, champions will take what they deserve. They know how much was invested, and they understand that they are the most prepared. They paid their dues—they refuse to lose.

#55 The Mark Of A Champion

Turning weaknesses into strengths is the mark of a champion. It may be easier and more fun to practice what you already do well, but that won't do much for improving your game. Champions make a habit of spending the majority of their practice time working on their weaknesses. If you're going to compete with the best, don't practice like the rest.

WINNING WAYS

#56 Think Feedback, Not Setback

Feel your losses, but don't feel defeated. If you can't feel the pain from a loss, you can't experience the joy of victory. Take a loss to heart but keep it in perspective. Champions are known more for how they handle their losses than their wins. A loss will always hurt, but it should never make you feel like giving up. Look at it as only a lesson, not a final exam. Sometimes losses are necessary. They help you figure out what doesn't work. A loss should be perceived as feedback, not setback.

#57 Learn To End Up In First

It's harder to hold the lead than it is to come from behind. When you're behind, you have nothing to lose. You can gamble and let it all hang out. Never underestimate a person who has nothing to lose. When you're in the lead it's a different story. You have the burden of keeping up the intensity. Although you want to start congratulating yourself, you can't let down—you must not allow your mind to drift. All the pressure is on the leader. When you become one, stay focused, and you'll learn to end up as one.

#58 F.I.R.S.T.

F.I.R.S.T. (For Individuals Reflecting Superior Toughness)

First place is reserved for those who get it done in tough times. The competition for the top spot is stiff, but the ones who possess the winning combination of confidence and pride believe that the top spot is reserved for them. When the game gets tough, it's the ones who stay strong when others go weak who win. It's the one who possesses superior toughness who finishes first.

#59 Play To Win

When you get the lead, don't change your game, don't let up, and don't become too conservative. If you're going to win, you must maintain the mental hustle that got you there. Keep the game face on. The momentum will change quickly if your opponent senses a letdown. Keep the pressure up but don't over pursue. Stay on your toes and off your heels. Protect the lead but look to score. Play to win. Never play not to lose.

WINNING WAYS

#60 Quality Practice

It's not the time you put in, but what you put into the time that matters. Quality practice—that's how you improve. You must practice the way you plan on playing during a game. Bring the same intensity, the same enthusiasm. You can't expect to get better if you just go through the motions. It's in practice where you develop game toughness. It's where you develop an instinct for the game. It's where you develop the habits that lead to success.

#61 Winning Is A Mind-set

Think like a winner and you'll become a winner. Look for ways to get the job done, not reasons why you can't. Winners form the habit of doing the things that losers don't like to do. Winners visualize the rewards of success. Losers picture the penalties of failure. Winning is a mind-set—you either develop it or you don't.

#62 Second Best Is For The Rest

Some people always seem to win; they always seem to come out on top. When it comes down to the wire, they always have the desire. They have developed a level of pride that won't let them lose something that could easily be theirs. They refuse to settle for second best. They refuse to be like the rest. People aren't born winners, they develop into winners.

#63 The Big Mistakes

It's not always the great plays that win the game as much as it is the big mistakes that cost a victory. If you can cut back on making crucial mistakes, if you can stop shooting yourself in the foot, it's as good as adding a new weapon to your arsenal. The best way to cut back on your mistakes is to constantly visualize yourself doing things correctly. Practice preventing the big mistakes as much as you practice performing the great plays. Learn from your mistakes; learn not to make them.

WINNING WAYS

#64 Success Is Earned

Achieving success is no accident. Nobody stumbles onto success. It's one of those things that requires preparation, hard work, and perseverance. Some people always seem to be successful. They always seem to have all the luck. But the truth is they put in the time, spent the energy, and took the risk. There is no accident about it—success is earned.

#65 Program Yourself

When it comes to sports skills, your body works like a computer. In practice you program your skills, and on game day you need the right command to bring out the very best of what you have programmed. While you're playing, don't dwell on the past and don't try to predict the future. Stay in the moment, focus on what's happening right before your eyes—that is the command that will release what is stored.

MOTIVATION

#66 The Opportunity Of Summer
#67 L.O.S.E.R.
#68 No Luck About It
#69 You Have To Risk
#70 "Can't" Never Achieved Anything
#71 Don't Label Yourself
#72 Pre-Game Pep "Self" Talk
#73 They're Out There
#74 You May Be A Late Bloomer
#75 It Takes Courage
#76 It's Worse Than Losing
#77 Keep The Streak Going
#78 Could Of—Should Of

#66 The Opportunity Of Summer

Seize your summer. Be the one to come back the most improved player. Brew your skills all summer long, and when you show up for the season—blow in like a hurricane. Pour your heart into your workouts. Give yourself a real opportunity to blossom. This summer be the storm brewing on the horizon.

MOTIVATION

#67 L.O.S.E.R.

L.O.S.E.R. (Lack Of Staying Emotionally Revved)

Winners stay charged up—they never let up the intensity until it's over. From somewhere deep down comes the inner strength to keep them fired up until they have what they're after. They just can't seem to let go. They're turned on the entire time they are competing. Winners keep the pedal to the medal—they stay emotionally revved.

#68 No Luck About It

People who work hard always seem to be luckier. They always seem to be in the right place at the right time. The truth is they create their own luck. They're masters of their own fates. When opportunities pop up, they're always in a position to seize them. Chance will always play a part in everything you do, but if you work hard, chances are in your favor.

MOTIVATION

#69 You Have To Risk

Anybody can be a nobody, but it takes a strong person to be a somebody. It takes courage to achieve greatness. You have to put yourself to the test. You have to take risks, and when things become difficult, you have to stay strong in your attempt. You may bend but not break. To be somebody isn't for everybody.

#70 "Can't" Never Achieved Anything

"Can't" is not part of the vocabulary of winners. You create your own barriers, and set your own limitations. "I can't," never accomplished anything. "I will try," has produced wonders. When you turn your attention inward, listen to the part of you that is saying, "I can." You have to believe to achieve.

MOTIVATION

#71 Don't Label Yourself

You are not bound by your past. The limitations you experienced in the past are no indication of what you can accomplish now. The past is the past. With hard work and desire, you can improve anything. Believe in yourself—don't label yourself. What you couldn't do yesterday is always possible today.

#72 Pre-Game Pep "Self" Talk

Before every game, give yourself a pre-game pep talk: "I've worked hard and I put in the time. I belong here. I deserve to compete, I have paid the price. I love challenges and I love to play. I'm pumped and I'm ready to have fun." An athlete who is truly ready to play doesn't need to jump up and down and yell and scream to get excited; he or she is already motivated from within.

MOTIVATION

#73 They're Out There

You're not alone. Although only a few in your school have the internal drive and dedication that you possess, there is no need to feel alone; there are many more athletes like you everywhere. If all the high school students in the country were put into one big school, that school would be loaded with determined students like you.

#74 You May Be A Late Bloomer

Dig deeper. You have more ability than you think, you just haven't discovered it yet. Everyone has gifts, but without good work habits and perseverance, not everyone goes on to realize them. Don't sell yourself short before giving yourself a real chance. You may be a late bloomer. Just like a flower, without proper care you'll never fully blossom.

MOTIVATION

#75 It Takes Courage

Do you have the courage to make a real commitment? Committing to your best doesn't require much more of your free time, but it does require more quality time. You can make a commitment to sports and still have your school work your top priority. Everybody has the time for commitments but not everybody has the courage to commit the energy.

#76 It's Worse Than Losing

Don't be afraid to lose. If you have the courage to attempt, you have nothing to lose. Winning and losing are the outcomes. Attempting is what it's all about. The consequences of losing will never outweigh the rewards of your attempt. What's worse than losing is not giving it a shot, not competing at all.

MOTIVATION

#77 Keep The Streak Going

You're only a champion for a day. When you finally win it all, get ready to defend the title because the next day they're coming after you. You worked too hard to be one and done. Celebrate and cherish the win but don't let down, don't become satisfied. Mentally prepare to repeat. Keep the streak going. Create a dynasty. You're not going to continue to get things done if you spend all your time looking at your reflection in your trophy.

#78 Could Of—Should Of

Average athletes seldom achieve their potential. Average work ethics, average desire, and average practice habits all prevent them from tapping into their best. Their athletic genetics will remain unexplored territory, never to be fully discovered. They might not have become the best, but they could have been much better. They will join the long line of would of—could of—and should of's.

IN CONTROL

#79 G.U.T.S.
#80 A Seasoned Veteran
#81 Pressure Can Be A Good Thing
#82 The Magic Is In The Air
#83 Be The Calm That Settles The Sea
#84 Sports Rituals
#85 The Cream Rises To The Top
#86 Cage The Rage

#79 G.U.T.S.

G.U.T.S. (Great Under Tough Situations)

When the game heats up, do you rise to the occasion? When crunch time nears, do you demand the ball—do you yearn for the spotlight? When the game is on the line, do you step forward when others around you shy away? When it's time to perform under pressure, do you perform at your best? If this doesn't sound like you, start treating every moment in practice like it were the big moment in a game, and you too, will develop GUTS.

IN CONTROL

#80 A Seasoned Veteran

Athletes who mentally prepare for competition rarely choke in the big games. The days preceding a big event, picture yourself performing with ease in every pressure situation you could possible face on game day. Create the entire scene in your mind. Picture the very atmosphere. Take the time and energy to visualize yourself performing in the clutch and you'll come through like a seasoned veteran on game day.

#81 Pressure Can Be A Good Thing

Thrive on pressure situations. Allow them to bring out your best. Pressure should be a positive thing—something that makes you stronger, not stressed. If you have a positive outlook and a focused mind, a pressure situation gives you the edge. It helps you shine when the game is on the line. Under great pressure a piece of coal becomes a diamond.

IN CONTROL

#82 The Magic Is In The Air

Even great athletes get nervous and develop butterflies before competition. Butterflies are a natural and normal part of competing, but if you let them get the best of you, they can affect your performance right from the get go. When you start to feel them come on before the competition begins, sit down, clear your mind, and take five deep, slow breaths. As you exhale, sense your muscles letting go. Keep your mind quiet and focused only on your breathing, and the butterflies will slowly disappear…the magic is in the air.

GYMBAG WISDOM—106 Ways To Become A Better Athlete

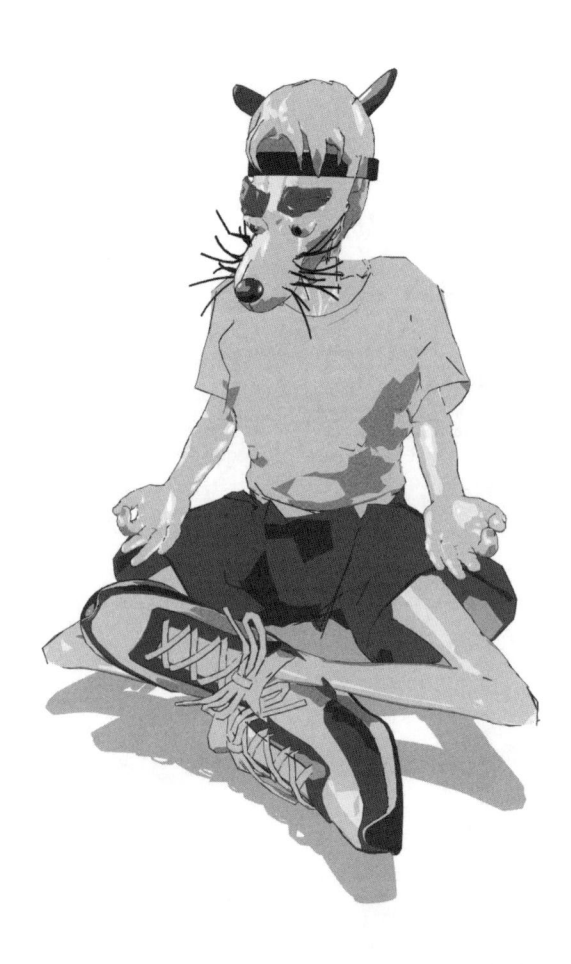

IN CONTROL

#83 Be The Calm That Settles The Sea

In the heat of the battle, be the one not to rattle. In the face of adversity, be the one to remain strong. When others are in need of emotional support, be the pillar of strength they can lean on. When others begin to unravel from the pressure, provide the inner strength to help hold them together. Be the calm that settles the sea.

#84 Sports Rituals

The next time you're watching sports on television, observe the simple sport rituals athletes go through before they perform. They help athletes prepare; they're part of their pre-performance routine. Rituals act as a starting point. They set a beat—one, two, three, and go. They help athletes get the momentum up and rolling step by step, and when the pressure builds and crunch time arrives, rituals help athletes remain focused, relaxed, and in the true state of competitive readiness.

IN CONTROL

#85 The Cream Rises To The Top

Focus on yourself. Direct your own destiny. Concern yourself with what's better for you and not with who's better than who. Keep your attention at home—concentrate on improving yourself. Focus on what you need to do to get better and not on the need to be better than someone else. The cream always rises to the top.

#86 Cage The Rage

Cage the rage. Before you fly off the handle, give yourself a little time to calm down. Get control of your temper before it controls you. When you feel an emotional overload coming on, stop and count to ten before you react. When you're in the heat of the moment, you have to keep your head—you have to maintain your composure to the very end. Losing your head can cost you the game…and sometimes it can cost you much more.

THE OLD FASHION WAY

#87 Be A Grizzly
#88 To Make Real Progress
#89 Self-Pride
#90 Push Yourself
#91 Adversity Will Make You Stronger
#92 No Fatigue Pain, No Gain

#87 Be A Grizzly

Work like a bear. When it's time to work out or practice, dig your claws in and make every minute count. On every repetition reach deep down inside for maximum effort. If you're going to make a commitment to a sport, make the commitment to bring high octane energy to every session. To really make big time progress, you have to attack your work furiously. If you're going to work like a bear—be a grizzly.

THE OLD FASHION WAY

#88 To Make Real Progress

You can't accomplish much if you work hard only on the days you feel great. Nobody feels a hundred percent every day, but the people who succeed give a hundred percent all the time. Build a tolerance for discomfort. To make real progress, to experience great things in life, you have to work through some discomfort. You have to give consistent effort no matter how you feel.

#89 Self-Pride

Have self-pride with an "attitude." Whatever you do, don't let anybody outwork you. It's one thing for somebody to beat you because they have more talent, but it's another thing to let somebody beat you because they have outworked you. When it comes to work ethic, everyone is on an equal playing field. A strong work ethic is the most important piece of the puzzle for success. There are many unsuccessful talented people out there walking the streets.

THE OLD FASHION WAY

#90 Push Yourself

When it's time to work out, work all out. If you're going to get stronger, you have to push yourself beyond your assumed limit. When you think you can't do another repetition, understand that is the rep that makes the difference—that is the one that makes you stronger. All the preceding reps just maintain what you already have. It's not the exercise, or the exercise program that makes the big difference, it's the effort that goes into whatever you do.

#91 Adversity Will Make You Stronger

When things don't go your way, learn to work even harder. Instead of retreating and getting down on yourself, keep your spirits up and increase the intensity. Successful people believe that no matter how many times things go wrong, there is plenty of time to make things go right. They have learned early on that adversity makes them stronger.

THE OLD FASHION WAY

#92 No Fatigue Pain, No Gain

Have you been to the edge? Have you pushed yourself to the outer limits of fatigue and not let up? If you don't consistently train on the edge, you will not improve your tolerance to fatigue pain. To gain strength and endurance, you need to overload your muscles. When fatigue is knocking on the door, stay focused on contracting your muscles and keeping your breathing deep and smooth. Don't let your mind drift to the pain—be mentally tough. If you push yourself to the limit, today's fatigue pain will become only tomorrow's discomfort. No fatigue pain, no gain.

CREATING THE WILL

#93 The "Eye Of The Tiger"
#94 Stoking The Fire
#95 Unravel The Mystery
#96 The Most Common Regret

CREATING THE WILL

#93 The "Eye Of The Tiger"

How does one develop the "eye of the tiger?" How does one create that deep-down desire to succeed? How does one develop a hunger for success? It all begins with understanding why you want to compete, why you want to excel. Think long and hard, then write down on paper your ten deepest reasons. Hang them on your bedroom mirror and review them and update them often—create an ongoing appetite for success. If you work hard you will improve, when you improve you will develop pride. The more you improve, the more pride you'll gain. Pride is behind the eye of the tiger.

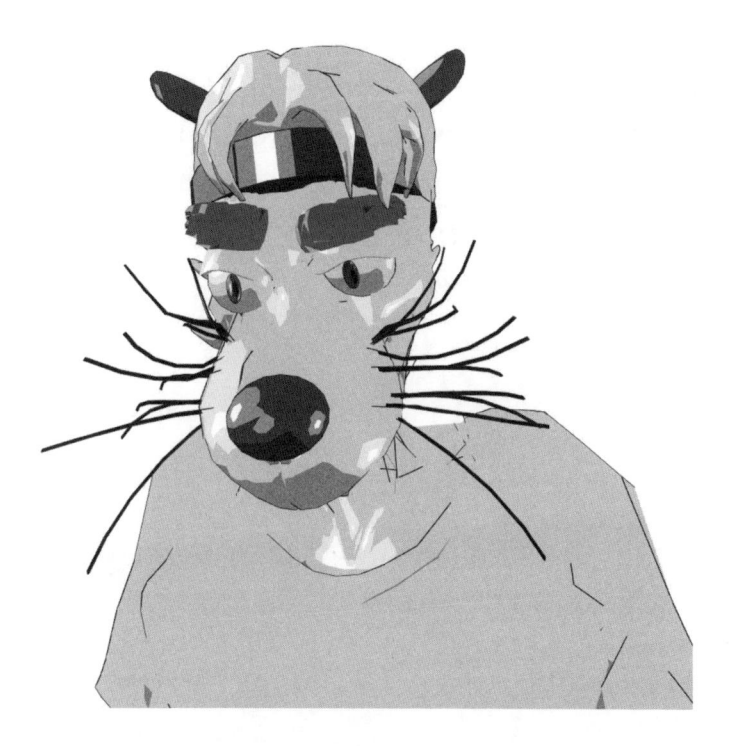

GYMBAG WISDOM—106 Ways To Become A Better Athlete

CREATING THE WILL

#94 Stoking The Fire

Make practicing like brushing your teeth. Something you just do automatically everyday, hopefully twice a day. Once you're in a routine you won't have to create energy every day for practice, because it will become a habit. It will show up automatically. Your energy level is the result of your state of mind.

#95 Unravel The Mystery

You're on your way, just continue to play. If you're any good at something, you know you can get better. You can sense it—you can taste it. Deep down you feel the urge to take it to the next level. Now it's a matter of having the pride, the curiosity, to push yourself to the limit. There is a natural desire to unravel the mystery of what's hidden in your genetic make-up—don't resist it.

CREATING THE WILL

#96 The Most Common Regret

Time flies. Your scholastic sports career will be over before you know it. Although it may feel like an eternity until you graduate, in the end it will seem as if your sports career went by in dog years. Work hard and improve now, because later comes sooner than you think. One of the most common regrets mumbled by recent graduates: "If only I had one more year."

SUPPORT SYSTEMS

#97 Be Coachable
#98 Pack Of Wolves
#99 Give Thanks
#100 Building Team Spirit

SUPPORT SYSTEMS

#97 Be Coachable

Always remain coachable. Always be ready for advice. Even if you think you have it all together, listen to what coaches have to say. Always keep an open mind and a receptive ear to constructive criticism. Sometimes you become so comfortable with what you're doing, you can't believe that you're doing things incorrectly. Never become set in your ways; conquer your resistance to change. A successful athlete is a coachable athlete.

#98 Pack Of Wolves

Showcase your talents, but within the constraints of the team. Individual effort can never outperform the team. A team playing as one unit has a collective focus, a combined force—it's members share a common goal. Together they can accomplish more. Teamwork is when everybody plays a role and nobody plays out of control. In the wild, a wolf doesn't stand a chance alone, but when it teams up with the pack, it's nearly unbeatable.

SUPPORT SYSTEMS

#99 Give Thanks

The next time a parent or guardian gives you a ride to or from practice, make sure you thank them. Rather than taking them for granted, show a little appreciation. They're not giving you a ride because they owe you something. They're giving you a ride to provide support. It's hard to reach your goals when you don't have support from the important people in your life.

#100 Building Team Spirit

Take time to give back. Remember how it felt when an older teammate took the time to help you out. Remember what it did for you. Give a younger athlete a lift. Help him raise his game to a higher level. That's what team pride is all about—that's how you can give back to the program—that's how school tradition is built. And understand also that coaching what you were taught is great review for yourself.

SUPPORT SYSTEMS

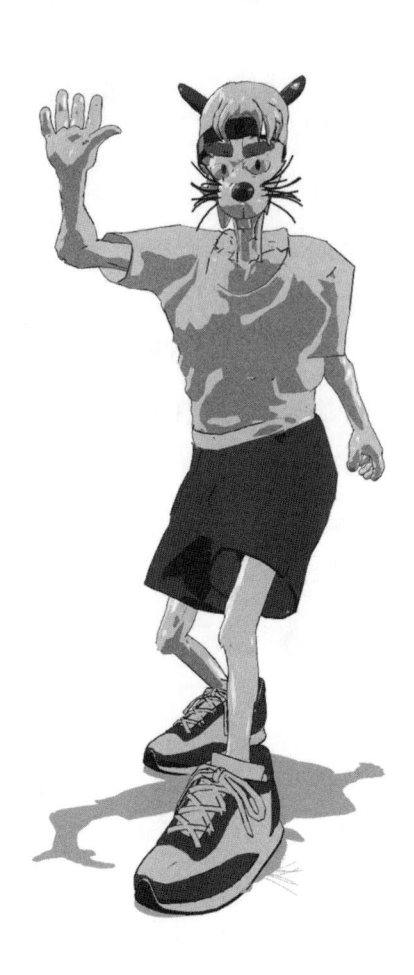

LOCKER ROOM WRAP-UP

#101 May The Force Be With You
#102 Keep Your Head Up
#103 The Big Lie
#104 Feel Like A Champion
#105 The Golden Sports Rule
#106 It's Not The Size Of The Trophy

LOCKER ROOM WRAP-UP

#101 May The Force Be With You

When it isn't fun anymore it's time to hang up the cleats. Only when you play for the fun of it will you experience more success. A superstar professional athlete was once asked to share his secret to his continuing success. He replied that he never went to work, he just went to play. Fun is energizing—it is the driving force that keeps you coming back. Fun links you to your higher power. When you take the fun out of sports you lose the force.

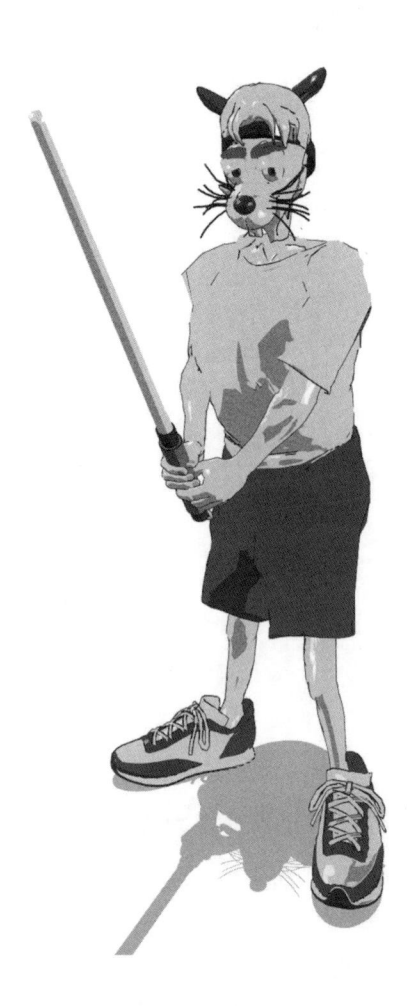

GYMBAG WISDOM—106 Ways To Become A Better Athlete

LOCKER ROOM WRAP-UP

#102 Keep Your Head Up

Keep your head up. Athletes who commit themselves entirely rarely hang their heads in defeat. They know they did all they could to prepare, and that is all anybody can ask. If you paid the price, even in defeat, you will be proud to walk with your head held high. But if you tried shortcuts, it will feel natural to let your head hang.

#103 The Big Lie

Steroids are a big lie. They don't make you a better athlete, just a heavier one. There are no short cuts to success. Nothing replaces hard work and dedication. Steroids in any form are extremely dangerous. It's hard to grasp the long-term effects when you're living in the short term, but when it comes to steroids you must think ahead, or you may end up dead…way before your time.

LOCKER ROOM WRAP-UP

#104 Feel Like A Champion

A big prize lies within the journey. Chase your dreams, but make sure you enjoy the ride. There are many personal achievements and triumphs along the way. As you pursue your goals, learn to cherish the little victories. You don't have to wait for your dreams to come true to feel like a champion.

#105 The Golden Sports Rule

Be a gracious winner. Embrace the golden sports rule; in victory, do unto your opponents as you would want them to do unto you. Celebrate with your teammates, not in the face of your opponents. True winners respect their competitors. Keep in mind that you were better than they only that day…and there will be other days.

LOCKER ROOM WRAP-UP

#106 It's Not The Size Of The Trophy

What does the gold medal stand for? It's such a small award for such a big event. Why? Because the real reward of the Olympics is achieved before any medal is handed out. The real reward is discovering what it takes just to make it to the Olympics. The gold medal signifies that sports aren't just about finishing first, but more about commitment, dedication, perseverance, and the pursuit of excellence. It's not the size of the trophy, but the size of the experience that matters.

GYMBAG WISDOM—106 Ways To Become A Better Athlete

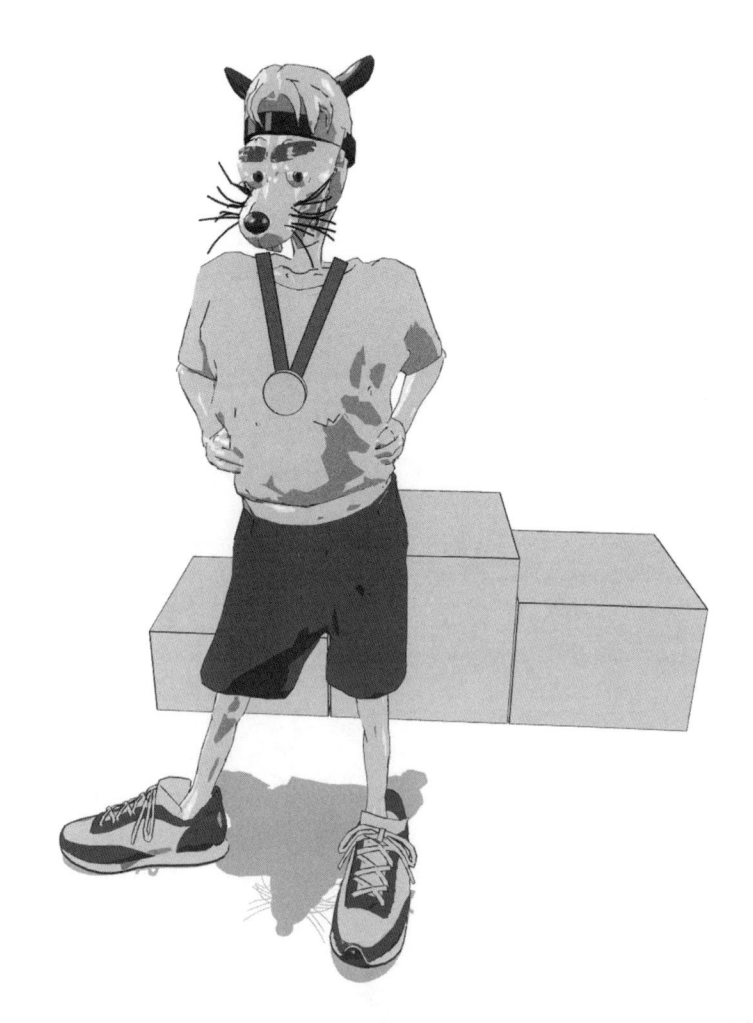

*For more information
about Gymbag Wisdom
visit:* **GymbagWisdom.com**
or call: **1-800-431-1579**

*For additional copies of Gymbag Wisdom,
check your local bookstore or order:*

By Telephone
1-800-431-1579

By Internet
Visit www.GymbagWisdom.com

By Mail
*ZonePress
P.O. Box 1778, Doylestown, PA 18901*

Make checks payable to ZonePress.

*$14.95 plus $1.95 for shipping and handling.
($0.95 S&H for each additional book)*

Special bulk orders available.